Limbic-predominant Age-related TDP-43 Encephalopathy

Late (The Newest Dementia)

BELLER HEALTH

This book is dedicated to people diagnosed with LATE, and their loved ones.

CONTENTS

ACKNOWLEDGMENTS

Thanks to the Atlanta Center for Medical Research, Stanford Medicine, Harvard Medical School, Emory Hospital, Alzheimer's Association, the National Institute on Aging, Alzheimer's Disease Center, Alzheimer's Foundation of America, the Mayo Clinic, Duke University Medical Center, Stanford Library School of Medicine, the National Library of Medicine, Johns Hopkins Medical, National Institutes of Health, and several other organizations that provided information used for this book. Thanks to everybody who assisted this book, everybody at Alzheimer's & Dementia Research Institute (ADRI). To my editor, John Briggs, who helps me improve every book. To all sources and for the photos. Most of all, thanks to my wife, Nicola Beller.

FOREWORD

Before we begin *LATE (Limbic-predominant age-related TDP-43 encephalopathy)*, let's review the series.

The <u>Dementia Risk Factors, Symptoms, Diagnosis, Stages, Treatment, Prevention Series</u> devotes a book to each dementia.

The series is organic, meaning it is an evolving work, and each book receives major annual updates. As science uncovers information, we add the important data in new editions.

The series also differentiates from most medical books because I write in everyday language. We might describe the writing goal in two ways:

1. Simplify the language where nonscientists and those outside the medical profession can comprehend.
2. Honor the science and facts, and the best scientists, researchers, and health professionals.

The series focuses a spotlight on dementias with no cure, nor accurate testing.

The books:

Dementia Risk Factors, Symptoms, Diagnosis, Stages, Treatment, Prevention, Prevention Series

Alzheimer's Risk Factors & Symptoms

Behavioral Variant Frontotemporal Dementia (bvFTD)

Primary Progressive Aphasia (PPA)

Dementia with Lewy Bodies

Parkinson's disease

Huntington's Disease

Normal Pressure Hydrocephalus

Wernicke-Korsakoff Syndrome

LATE (Limbic-predominant age-related TDP-43 encephalopathy)

Among the worst news we can hear is that we or one of our loved ones has dementia. A killer disease with no cure pumps fear in the bravest souls.

I have witnessed how this medical condition destroys, not just the inflicted person, but their loved ones. Besides the patient, nobody suffers more than voluntary caregivers.

If I had a magic wand, I would wipe away the pain.

Instead, I study dementia year around to write and release annual updates.

Who is the reading audience?

The audience for this series falls in five categories.

Those diagnosed with dementia

If medical authorities diagnose you with dementia, my heart goes out to you. You're in for a long battle, and you want to slow the disease and extend the quality of life as long as possible.

Loved ones of those diagnosed

If your loved one has a dementia, he or she needs you. Depending on the type, the dementia causes behavioral problems, memory issues, motor decline, and other psychological and physical disorders. The learning curve is fast and changes as one moves from one stage to the next.

Medical professionals interested in a dementia overview

If you are a medical professional interested in a quick elementary lesson on Dementia, this is a good option.

Volunteer & professional caregivers

If you are a dementia caregiver, you are also in for a long difficult march. Dementia patients demand 24/7 care in later stages, requiring help going to the bathroom, bathing, and with other basic daily functions.

Anybody interested in learning about a disease that strikes 1 of 6 Americans, and 1

of 3 seniors

This series is a good option for anybody who wants to gain a basic understanding of the 16 dementias.

While dementia is a scary disease, the series is not frightening. The books include the facts and science as they exist at the time of this writing.

As much as possible, we replace medical jargon with everyday language.

These books are a straightforward conversation warm and friendly.

Series First Lesson

Nothing I say or write should replace a competent doctor. Doctors, much like teachers, are part of a sacred profession.

While informal education is a lifetime pursuit, formal education is crucial. I detest the worst teachers, for they let down students and society, but I love and respect the best teachers, true pillars of society.

I also abhor incompetent, greedy doctors who let down their patients and society, but love and respect the best. A wise course for the profession is to weed out incompetent, uncaring, corrupt doctors and medical professionals. The medical profession also should listen to and follow the best within their profession. The worst thing we can do is pretend all doctors (or any profession) are the same.

Nothing good I write about the medical profession includes incompetent, uncaring doctors, nurses, etc. And nothing bad I write about the medical profession includes the best.

Like when picking a school, you want one in the upper fifty percent, the same is true for medical facilities and doctors.

Although the series criticizes the profession when deserved, the first lesson in this series is *find a competent doctor*. If you have one, count your blessings. If you do not, find one.

A bad doctor is nothing more than a glorified idiot, a dangerous parasite who dishonors a noble profession. These people are smart enough to get through medical school, but greedy or otherwise flawed beyond redemption. A doctor who does not care for his or her patients is worse than worthless.

At some point, Big pharmaceuticals, Big Insurance, and their political puppets appointed doctors sanctioned drug dealers, the worse little or no better than those on the worst corners.

Find a competent, dedicated, caring, experienced, informed doctor who listens and respects your opinion, and writes prescriptions as a LAST RESORT.

I offer the same advice in all my health books. Without the right doctor, you are at the mercy of a profit-oriented health system that seldom puts the patient's interests first, second, or third.

However, nothing I say or write in these books or elsewhere means you should not see a doctor, should stop taking your medication, or otherwise undermine the medical profession's ability to diagnose and treat any medical symptoms you might experience.

What I want you to do is find a good doctor you trust with your life and ask him or her pointed questions concerning your health and any treatment they recommend.

How many dementias?

Not counting mixed dementia, there are sixteen primary dementia types:

1. Alzheimer's disease

Lewy body dementia

2. Dementia with Lewy bodies/DLB
3. Parkinson's disease dementia/PDD

Vascular dementia

4. Buerger's disease
5. Intestinal ischemic syndrome
6. Peripheral artery disease
7. Popliteal entrapment syndrome
8. Raynaud's phenomenon
9. Renal artery disease

Frontotemporal dementia (FTD)

10. Behavioral Variant Frontotemporal Dementia (bvFTD)
11. Primary Progressive Aphasia (PPA)

Other Dementias

12. Normal pressure hydrocephalus
13. Creutzfeldt-Jacob
14. Wernicke-Korsakoff
15. Huntington's disease
16. LATE (the newest dementia category)

17. *Mixed dementia

*Not a specific dementia, but a combination, mixed dementia is the seventeenth category important in any dementia discussion.

Any disease leading to dementia symptoms is a dementia type, but the 16 listed represent most cases.

The series teaches the basics for each dementia. You will learn certain patterns. While there are no known cures and these diseases are irreversible, we control many of the habits causing dementia.

While genetics, age, and luck play a role in dementia, like most diseases, most cases result from unhealthy habits.

We are not bashing those victimized by genetics and age, but most people own the ability to avoid or postpone dementia.

For instance, those who use tobacco and abuse alcohol skyrocket their chances of dementia, including Alzheimer's disease. You will learn how healthier habits increase your chances of never getting or slowing the dreadful disease.

Dementia is costly, deadly, and in most cases avoidable. The disease terrifies, but we are not helpless. A good defense is the best solution to any formidable offense, and in the fight to remain healthy, our best defense is developing the healthy lifestyle advocated in this book.

I do not promise you a miracle cure. Nor does financial gain guide my mission, but hopes of helping others.

I am a researcher, nutritionist, and author, and witnessed Alzheimer's disease, and other dementias invade, destroy and kill loved ones. This series on dementia and Alzheimer's provides the average person around the world easy-to-learn books covering complicated medical subjects.

I will challenge the medical profession where necessary, just as in my political books I criticize Congress and the

United States government for their mistakes or shortcomings.

Not that I am smarter than the average doctor or politician, but I offer a perspective those inside the medical bubble cannot.

My brief career as a Congressional staffer taught me how difficult it is to maintain one's focus inside the bubble. Seeing the big picture is no less challenging inside the medical bubble motivated by profit.

Profiteers and those wanting to credit or discredit somebody funds too many studies to promote their own product or discredit somebody else's.

This book series holds no ulterior agenda. The small royalty fees are the only compensation. I have accepted no money from corporations to promote their product, nor do I have an ax to grind with anybody in the medical profession.

I hold a profound respect for ethical, competent, dedicated, and hardworking nurses, doctors, and other medical personnel. Nor is there anything wrong when medical-related businesses — including hospitals, pharmaceutical companies, and insurance companies — make a reasonable profit for worthy medical supplies and services. But, I detest those who inflate prices for desperate people, or are incompetent.

My goal is to provide you a simple, short, informational guide so you can understand the different dementias, their symptoms, and causes before it strikes your family. Dementia kills one out of every six Americans. No family, no matter how wealthy, no matter where located, no matter their race, no matter their educational level is immune from dementia.

I hope dementia never strikes your family.

Because dementia attacks one of six families, I wrote this

series to help you prepare (as much as possible) for the 16 dementias.

As the series name suggests, each book covers symptoms, causes, diagnosis, treatment, stages, and prevention for dementia covered.

The text contains American and British English. I write in American English, but the research comes from the best studies worldwide. Therefore, quotes from British, Australian, and some other researchers are in British English. For integrity, I do not edit quotes.

Having explained the series, let's focus on *LATE (Limbic-predominant age-related TDP-43 encephalopathy)*. Chapter one provides a basic overview.

Chapter 1: LATE (Limbic-predominant age-related TDP-43 encephalopathy)?

We proposed a new name to increase recognition and research for this common cause of dementia, the symptoms of which mimic Alzheimer's dementia but is not caused by plaques and tangles (the buildup of beta amyloid proteins that Alzheimer's produces). Rather, LATE dementia is caused by deposits of a protein called TDP-43 in the brain.

—Julie Schneider[1]

What is LATE (Limbic-predominant age-related TDP-43 encephalopathy)?

The latest classified dementia, LATE is similar enough to have been misdiagnosed as Alzheimer's until international researchers confirmed, named, and explained the new dementia in the April 2019 edition of the journal *Brain*.

An international team including researchers Australia, Austria, Japan, Sweden, United Kingdom, United States, and elsewhere named and defined a new dementia type, *LATE*[2] *(Limbic-predominant age-related TDP-43 encephalopathy).*

Nina Silverberg[3], PhD., Director of the NIA Alzheimer's Disease Centers and Richard J. Hodes[4], M.D., director of the National Institute on Aging (NIA) co-chaired the workshop in Atlanta[5] in October 2018. They released their study's results in the journal *Brain* in April 2019; their findings making us reevaluate much of what we have believed about Alzheimer's and the broader category, dementia.

This book provides a basic overview of this new dementia category. We will expand the book as new studies on LATE emerge, but use all available to describe a dementia condition previously classified as Alzheimer's.

Right and wrong, people call dementia the "old folks' disease." While most dementia strikes seniors, some types strike infants as young as two. Study results show our topic, LATE (Limbic-predominant age-related TDP-43 encephalopathy) definitely qualifies as a geriatrics medical condition.

One of four people over 85 have enough TDP-43 buildup to cause cognitive decline, executive function deterioration, and memory loss[6].

According to Robert Howard, a professor of old age psychiatry at University College London, the consensus work study results are "probably the most important paper to be published in the field of dementia in the last five years[7]."

"Those of us who work in dementia have long been puzzled by our patients who have all the symptoms of Alzheimer's disease, but whose brains do not contain the pathological features of the condition," said Howard. "We now know that these puzzling patients are probably suffering from LATE and not Alzheimer's disease and that LATE may be 'mimicking' Alzheimer's in about 20% of cases."

In this chapter, we define the latest recognized dementia, LATE (Limbic-predominant age-related TDP-43 encephalopathy).

Several researchers the past couple of decades pointed towards TDP-43 and suggested a new dementia type.

The first pathological recognition of LATE occurred in a 1994 study when researchers discovered 13 patients had the then-unnamed dementia. The study represents the first documented account of LATE.

Researchers and the medical community continued to notice, study, and document LATE for 25 years until April 2019 when the National Institute of Health sponsored international group of researchers named, classified, and described the disease.

"People have, in their own separate bailiwicks, found different parts of the elephant," said Dr. Peter Nelson. "But this is the first place where everybody gets together and says, 'This is the whole elephant[8].'"

Dr. Nelson and dozens of research groups around the world collaborated over a decade on the groundbreaking project.

Another member, Melissa Murray, PhD., molecular neurologist from the Mayo Clinic explained their purpose: "develop diagnostic criteria for LATE, aiming both to stimulate research and to promote awareness of this pathway to dementia[9]."

Not Frontotemporal Lobar Degeneration or Amyotrophic Dementia!

The TDP-43 protein is also associated with frontotemporal lobar generation and amyotrophic lateral sclerosis, but LATE is a separate medical condition.

How Prevalent is LATE?

According to Dr. Peter Nelson, LATE is "disease that's 100 times more common than (ALS or FTLD), and nobody knows about it."

Nelson admits we do not yet know LATE's prevalence.

Data suggests LATE is rare for younger people, but as prevalent as Alzheimer's in the oldest members of our specie.

The international team of NIH sponsored researchers who named and defined LATE estimate 20-50% above age 80 demonstrate the LATE-related TDP unfolding[10].

BELLER HEALTH

Why is Categorizing LATE Important?

Bart De Strooper[11], molecular biologist, professor, University of London and the UK Dementia Research Institute explained the importance of the new dementia category:

1) "It will refocus attention to TDB-43 physiology and stimulate work to find biomarkers for this pathology so that we can make more refined diagnosis.
2) It explains possibly to a certain extent why some trials in the Alzheimer field failed: while they were curing the amyloid pathology, TDB-43 pathology just went on.
3) It will stimulate industry to find drugs against TDB-43 or related pathways[12]."

Peter Nelson Explaining the Working Group's Purpose

Working Group Cochair Peter Nelson[13] explained:

1. The consensus working group report on LATE was that — a distillation of what an international, multidisciplinary group could agree on.

*2. The goal was not to produce a trendy new term. For me personally, a key goal was to have a diagnosis that could be made in a meaningful way. For example, at our center, we just signed out nine cases and four demonstrated what I can now call LATE-NC. It is not meaningful (or rather, it is needlessly puzzling) to patients, clinicians, or anybody else when different diagnosticians apply completely different terms and criteria for a **common phenomenon. The best e-mail I got in the past few days was from a respected colleague who wrote, "I already used LATE as a diagnosis today!"***

3. This was not a paper about FTD/FTLD. The commonalities and differences related to LATE-NC and FTLD-TDP were, naturally, a point of discussion among the group. Without getting down in the weeds, a consensus was not reached on that. Here are some differences that were agreed on and are highlighted in the paper: LATE-NC is ~100-fold more prevalent than FTLD-TDP (lifetime risk is 1:4 versus ~1:1000);

LATE-NC tends to affect people in a quantumly older age group; persons with FTLD-TDP tend to have language and/or behavioral differences that have not been described in LATE; rather, persons with LATE-NC at autopsy tended to have deficits in episodic memory. I, personally, would guess that those differences will be shown to be correlated with differences in the neuropathology, and other parameters, but time will tell. MAPT haplotypes make all sorts of tauopathies worse; doesn't make them all FTLD-Tau. Just as not all tauopathies are AD, not all TDP-43 proteinopathies are FLTD/ALS.

4. This is a massively underappreciated and understudied disease(s) – and yes, TDP-43 proteinopathy (with or without comorbid AD pathology) is strongly associated with cognitive impairment, although, for a gradually progressive disease that affects >85-year-olds preferentially, a lot of persons die in a presumed preclinical state.

It is of course true that this is not the first word on age-related TDP-43 proteinopathy, nor, of course, the last. However, this is the first consensus group effort to address this topic, and it is hoped that this paper will help to move the field forward.

Peter Nelson wrote the above quote in Alzheimer's Forum in response to a thorough review, and comments by other researchers.

Several international researchers participated in the lively discussion. LATE is a hot topic within the medical community. I applaud Nelson and his colleagues for their ground shaking report.

Will future studies change some work group consensus findings, advance other theories, and address issues the work group did not?

I hope so!

Nelson and his distinguished colleagues did not present their findings as the final LATE or TDP-43 statement, but instead provide a framework to address a widespread dementia previously misdiagnosed. Again, well done!

Because of the work group's consensus, science can evolve and address the unanswered questions. The work group's findings provide researchers a framework to finally study LATE as a separate disease from Alzheimer's.

Which brings us to an appropriate question: When is Alzheimer's not Alzheimer's?

Chapter 2: When is Alzheimer's LATE?

Since LATE (Limbic-predominant age-related TDP-43 encephalopathy) has been misdiagnosed for Alzheimer's until the reclassification, this chapter focuses on the distinction between the two dementias.

Researchers predict the medical profession misdiagnosed hundreds of thousands of people with LATE as Alzheimer's disease, meaning they administered the wrong medications and treatment[14].

Richard J. Hodes, M.D., director of the National Institute on Aging (NIA) addresses a question many researchers and doctors ask.

"While we've certainly been making advances in Alzheimer's disease research — such as new biomarker and genetic discoveries — we are still at times asking, 'When is Alzheimer's disease not Alzheimer's disease in older adults?" said Hodes. "The guidance provided in this report, including the definition of LATE, is a crucial step toward increasing awareness and advancing research for both this disease and Alzheimer's as well."

LATE "mimics" Alzheimer's but they are different diseases.

Difference between LATE and Alzheimer's

Alzheimer's and LATE share similar symptoms but not pathologies.

Mutated TDP-43 protein unfolding causes LATE, whereas beta amyloid protein plaques and tau tangles cause Alzheimer's[15]. Different proteins are responsible for the two dementia types, and the deposits form in different regions of the brain.

In Alzheimer's, the amyloid protein and neurofibrillary (tau) tangles attack hippocampus and entorhinal cortex in the beginning, and later the cerebral cortex[16]. In the beginning, Alzheimer's attacks memory, while later causing declines in reasoning, language, and social behavior[17].

In LATE, the TDP-43 protein misfolds in the amygdala brain region and causes episodic memory loss in the beginning. In middle stages, the protein forms in the hippocampus, and in late stage in the middle frontal gyrus, which causes cognitive decline[18].

Diagnosing LATE is difficult because it and Alzheimer's share symptoms. If not for the differing causes, they would be the same dementia. But, they have different protein sources and are different dementias.

We have far to go in diagnosing Alzheimer's and LATE, but especially the latter. Researchers and doctors have been developing the pathology for Alzheimer's for decades, whereas the science behind LATE's pathology remains in its infancy.

To know with certainty somebody has LATE, medical authorities must conduct an autopsy. This remains the unfortunate reality for many dementias.

We need better, cheaper means to diagnose LATE, Alzheimer's, and the other dementias. Dr Carol Routledge, Director of Research from Alzheimer's Research UK addressed the problem.

"People are diagnosed with a specific form of dementia based on the symptoms they experience," said Routledge. "When the symptoms of diseases overlap, it is very difficult to reliably determine the underlying cause[19]."

Although symptoms do not distinguish LATE from Alzheimer's, there are subtle hints. LATE develops slower than Alzheimer's disease[20], which provides contrast, if not clarity.

Can Somebody have LATE and Alzheimer's at the same time?

There is a dementia category called "mixed dementia" because multiple dementias are often present at once.

LATE and Alzheimer's are sometimes both present, and when this happens, the symptoms grow faster and are more devastating[21].

How does LATE change the way we view Alzheimer's?

Nina Silverberg, PhD., Director of the NIA Alzheimer's Disease Centers explained why the LATE dementia classification effects our outlook on Alzheimer's and dementia.

"Recent research and clinical trials in Alzheimer's disease have taught us two things: First, not all of the people we thought had Alzheimer's have it; second, it is very important to understand the other contributors to dementia," said Silverberg. "In the past many people who enrolled in clinical trials likely were not positive for amyloid. "Noting the trend in research implicating TDP-43 as a possible Alzheimer's mimic, a group of experts convened a workshop to provide a starting point for further research that will advance our understanding of another contributor to late life brain changes[22]."

Studies on the previously known dementias confirm most are often misdiagnosed as Alzheimer's. The classification of LATE as a dementia means all LATE cases have been misdiagnosed as Alzheimer's in the past.

While this inflated Alzheimer's disease numbers (and led to more Alzheimer's research funds than other dementias), LATE patients have skewed outcomes of Alzheimer's medication and treatment research.

Drug Studies

The consensus group believe including LATE patients in Alzheimer's drug studies perhaps skewed the results.

"LATE probably responds to different treatments than

AD, which might help explain why so many past Alzheimer's drugs have failed in clinical trials," said Dr. Peter Nelson. "Now that the scientific community is on the same page about LATE, further research into the 'how' and 'why' can help us develop disease-specific drugs that target the right patients[23]."

The consensus team recommends removing LATE patients from Alzheimer's drug trials, an encourages independent studies for each dementia.

Learning what is not Alzheimer's helps pinpoint real treatment options. Drugs to treat the Alzheimer's proteins might not work on LATE and, as Dr. Nelson suggested, explain why so many Alzheimer's drug trials fail.

Chapter 3: LATE CAUSES & RISK FACTORS

Although the science is still developing, we cover Late causes and risk factors in this chapter.

What is TDP-43?

When discussing Alzheimer's, LATE, or one of the other dementias, the topic turns to protein buildup, plaques, tangles, and similar descriptions.

Like the other proteins, TDP-43 serves a vital function. Something, however, scientists do not understand, causes the protein to buildup in some type of clumps, killing brain cells and tissue.

What is TDP-43's normal function?

Located in the cell nucleus,TDP-43 binds to DNA, regulates transcription, initiating the first step in protein production.

The Genetics Home Reference[24] describes TDP-43.

This protein can also bind to RNA, a chemical cousin of DNA, to ensure the RNA's stability. The TDP-43 protein is involved in processing molecules called messenger RNA (mRNA), which serve as the genetic blueprints for making proteins. By cutting and rearranging mRNA molecules in different ways, the TDP-43 protein controls the production of different versions of certain proteins. This process is known as alternative splicing. The TDP-43 protein can influence various functions of a cell by regulating protein production.

The TARDBP gene is particularly active (expressed) during early development before birth when new tissues are forming. Many of the proteins whose production is influenced by the

*TDP-43 protein are involved in nervous system
and organ development.*

TDP-43 serves a vital role in our development and health, so why is it implicated in LATE (Limbic-predominant age-related TDP-43 encephalopathy)?

What goes wrong?

TDP-43 becomes problematic when it misfolds. When TDP-43 misfolds, it causes impaired thinking and memory loss[25].

Genes Increasing LATE Risk

Researchers links five genes to higher LATE risk[26].

- ABCC9
- APOE
- GRN
- KCNMB2
- TMEM106B

Other Late Risk Factors

Any LATE risk factors list remains incomplete until further research.

- Age

Besides the gene connections, age is the one confirmed LATE risk factor. The researchers suspect LATE is a disease that manifests in people's eighties, so every year past eighty increases one's risk.

Considering 20-50% of people over 85 have LATE, age is an undeniable risk factor.

Chapter 4: LATE STAGES & SYMPTOMS

As the newest dementia, standards will remain in a flux for years.

However, researchers have studied TDP-43 for decades, linking it to frontotemporal lobar degeneration and ALS.

We will examine the three stage model (early, mid, and late).

Three-Stage Model

Early Stage LATE

The TDP-43 protein associated with LATE is restricted to the amygdala brain region in stage one or early stage.

Early Stage LATE Symptoms

- Episodic memory

Middle Stage LATE

TDP-43 spreads to the hippocampus brain and occipitotemporal region in stage two or middle stage.

Middle Stage LATE Symptoms

- Cognitive decline

Late Stage LATE

In late stage LATE, TDP-43 forms in the amygdala, hippocampus, and middle frontal gyrus, including the basal forebrain, inferior temporal cortex, insula, and the ventral striatum.

Late Stage LATE Symptoms

- Severe memory loss

- Severe cognitive decline

Stages Sources: Consensus Working Group Report[27], *Medical Xpress*[28], *Medical News Today*[29], Advisory Board[30], National Institute on Aging[31]

Chapter 5: LATE DIAGNOSIS

LATE is a new dementia and therefore scientists must develop diagnosis tools. Of the chapters in this book, we expect this one to go through the most updates.

We need immediate studies to create diagnosis tools for LATE, as is the case for most dementias. Like the acronym for the disease, science is late compared to the other dementias.

While researchers have known and researched TDP-43 for years, most until now was related to ALS or frontotemporal degeneration.

The NIH supported international research team[32] established the criteria for LATE when they named and described the disease. With more research, I expect the medical profession to modify the criteria, but the starting point is the consensus the NIH-backed international research team developed following their comprehensive review of the TDP-43 protein[33] and its relation to LATE.

Recommended LATE Diagnosis & Staging

The NIH backed international team recommend an "anatomically-based preliminary staging scheme" with the following hierarchy for routine autopsy workups[34]:

1. Amygdala.
2. Hippocampus.
3. Middle frontal gyrus.

The review showed LATE concentrates in the temporal lobe, but neuroimaging studies demonstrate LATE causes atrophy in the frontal cortex, medial temporal lobes, and elsewhere[35].

The consensus team also pointed to genetic studies implicating five genes to LATE[36]:

1. ABCC9
2. APOE
3. KCNMB2
4. LATE-NC: GRN
5. TMEM106B

While the genetic risks suggests LATE, Alzheimer's, and frontotemporal lobar degeneration have similar pathogenetic processes, it also reconfirmed LATE is a unique disease[37].

We need more Studies!

The consensus authors pressed for immediate and specific research[38]:

> *Large gaps remain in our understanding of LATE. For advances in prevention, diagnosis, and **treatment**, there is an urgent need for research focused on LATE, including in vitro and animal models. An obstacle to clinical progress is lack of diagnostic tools, such as biofluid or neuroimaging biomarkers, for ante-mortem detection of LATE. Development of a disease biomarker would augment observational studies seeking to further define the risk factors, natural history, and clinical features of LATE, as well as eventual subject recruitment for targeted therapies in clinical trials.*

The NIH-backed researchers deserve credit for recognizing, categorizing, collecting the important data from decades of studies, calling for more research, and providing hope for hundreds of thousands of people before misdiagnosed and maltreated for Alzheimer's.

We will update this chapter as soon as researchers discover better diagnosis tools.

Beller Health Recommendations for Quicker and more Accurate Diagnosis

- A blood or urine test to detect LATE.

- If a blood or urine test is not possible, we need better biomarkers for CAT scans, MRIs, SPECT, and more expensive alternatives.

- A quick but thorough education on the 16 primary dementias, including LATE, for primary physicians, nurses, other medical professionals, and the public.

- Provide the medical community the tools to diagnose and treat this fatal disease.

- Research to confirm this is an old folks disease. We won't know how many younger people get LATE until the same research is done on younger people as on seniors eighty and over.

Chapter 6: LATE TREATMENT

As with diagnosis, we need dozens of studies to better establish LATE symptoms, risk factors, and treatment.

The treatment thus far treats symptoms, but does little to slow the disease's progress. While no cure exists, a 2019 Laval University study offers promise.

Nanomedicine

A study released in *The Journal of Clinical Investigation* focused on eliminating TDP-43 buildup. While the study was on mice, and focused on ALS, Laval University researchers from Canada and France worked to reduce TDP-43 protein buildup.

The researchers used a new nanomedicine tool, single-chain antibodies. While others have used the new tool before, the team used a novel scFV antibody VH7Vk9 and targeted the TDP-43 RRM1 domain. They concluded[39]:

> *We demonstrated that virus-mediated delivery of VH7Vk9 in the CNS of transgenic mice expressing mutant hDP-43 succeeded in ameliorating cognitive and motor deficits as well as in reducing TDP-43 proteinopathy and neuroinflammatory changes.*

Lead researcher Jean-Pierre Julien, Faculty of Medicine, Laval University, explained the team's next goal. "We are now trying to develop an approach that would not require the use of viruses," said Julien. "Preliminary results suggest that specific antibodies injected directly into the cerebrospinal fluid could reduce the formation of aggregates of the protein in nerve cells[40]."

We need human studies to verify the technique works on humans but, if proven valid, the nanomedicine tool can elevate LATE treatment beyond medication and therapy to treat symptoms.

If TDP-43 unfolding is responsible for LATE, reducing the buildup should slow, perhaps reverse the neuro damage.

I expect nanomedicine to revolutionize the medical

profession, leading to treatments never imagined possible. The Canadian and French researchers collaboration might provide a major breakthrough in treating LATE and other pathological problems caused by mutated protein buildup in the brain.

Studies like this should evolve in the coming months and years, so I will update this book once or twice per year.

Chapter 7: MINIMIZE RISK OR SLOW LATE & THE OTHER 15 DEMENTIAS

Besides how cruel LATE is, the worst aspect might be disease is incurable. Therefore, it is crucial we build our own defense system and do our best to prevent or slow these and other devastating diseases.

We've developed a 12-point plan to reduce your risks of getting, or slowing if you already have LATE or one of the other dementias.

The principles are discussed in greater detail in <u>Be the Best You!</u>

12-Point Plan to Prevent or Slow LATE & other Dementias

1. Avoid or limit drinking to 1 drink per day (female adults) or 2 (male adults).
2. Do not smoke or otherwise use tobacco products.
3. Eat a balanced, whole food diet (avoiding processed food).
4. Exercise 4-7 times per week, manage weight and keep within healthy margins. Avoid belly fat.
5. Socialize and remain active.
6. Read and otherwise exercise your mind.
7. Follow the Golden Rule, avoid negativity, shine a light.
8. Manage and control blood pressure, blood sugar, & cholesterol.
9. Avoid or treat stress, anxiety, and depression.
10. Don't demand or expect prescription drugs for every symptom. Ask questions about side effects.
11. Find legitimate reasons to laugh more than the average person.
12. Remain hydrated and avoid sugary drinks.

Above is the short list, but you'll gain incredible benefits if you follow those 12 suggestions.

Balanced, whole food diet

Few things like health and exercise predict one's health. No matter one's gender, race, nation, demographics, if all we know is their diet and amount of exercise, we can predict if they are healthy or unhealthy.

If we know somebody smokes, we can predict health issues and symptoms they might experience based on how much tobacco they consume.

If somebody is obese, we can predict associated health issues like high blood pressure, diabetes, and several cardiovascular issues.

In contrast, if a doctor knows somebody eats a balanced whole food diet and exercises 30-60 minutes five to seven times per week, he or she knows this person has reduced their risks and increased their ability to fight or slow dementia.

The food you eat can be either the safest and most powerful form of medicine or the slowest form of poison. — Dr. Ann Wigmore

---

Is your diet a "powerful form of medicine" or a recipe to tedious suicide?

Balanced whole foods including Omega-3, vegetables, fruits, beans, nuts, berries (blueberries), carotenoids, genistein, tea (green), coffee (black), spinach, unfried fish (salmon), flax seeds, chia seeds, kale, whole grains, and resveratrol are among the specific foods that lower risk of dementia.

A *PubMed* study found coconut oil, fresh herbs and spices, red wine, and olive oil reduce dementia risk[41].

The table below is incomplete, but provides the best current science. I divided the table into three categories: 1) Bad foods that cause neurogeneration; 2) Foods that require more studies. 3) Good foods providing neuroprotection.

Bad Foods/Need more Studies/Good Foods

The table below shows confirmed bad foods on the left, and science-backed good foods on the right. In the middle are foods requiring more studies, although the arrows point towards the direction preliminary studies show.

Bad foods	Need more studies	Good foods
Dairy	MUFA→	Omega-3
High fructose corn syrup	←PUFA	Fresh Vegetables
	←Saturated Fat	Fresh Fruits
White sugar	Vitamin C→	Nuts (Walnuts, Cashews, Macadamia)
Trans fat	Vitamin D→	
	Vitamin E →	
	Riboflavin→	Berries (Blueberries)
	←Carbohydrates	Olive Oil
	←Meat	Coconut Oil
		Fresh herbs &

		spices
		Unfried fish
		(Wild caught Salmon)
		Tea
		Coffee
		Resveratrol
		Carotenoids
		Genistein

We need more studies to expand the list, but this provides a good roadmap to an anti-LATE, anti-dementia diet. Include as many of the proven neuroprotection foods — herbs, spices, teas, coffee, and supplements — in your diet as possible.

A whole food diet includes:

- Whole grains (no white or processed flour!)
- Vegetables
- Fruit
- Salmon (Free caught fish)
- Blueberries
- Green tea (or other unsweetened teas)

- Coffee (unsweetened)

Supplements

- Resveratrol

Exercise

Physical activity promotes cardiovascular health, enhances cognitive skills, and improves one's longevity chances.

Humans build strength through exercise. Muscles without exercise turn to fat, which we must carry around like a bowling ball bag (or two or three). As we become weaker, we must carry larger and larger loads (us). This increases our chances of:

- Physical injury
- Obesity
- High blood pressure
- Cardiovascular disease
- Strokes
- Dementia (including LATE)
- Parkinson's disease
- Other diseases and medical conditions

Exercising reduces the risks for all diseases and medical conditions listed. Exercise four to seven times per week.

The NIH's "Physical Activity Guidelines for Americans" summarizes the human costs.

About $117 billion in annual health care costs and about 10 percent of premature mortality are associated with inadequate physical activity (not meeting the aerobic key guidelines).

Health Benefits from Exercising

- Better sleep
- Cognitive function benefits
- Decrease cancer risks
- Decrease early mortality risk
- **Decrease dementia risk**
- Decrease diabetes risk
- Decrease stress
- Fewer fall-related injuries
- Greater physical ability and well-being
- Improves quality of life
- Improves physical ability
- Lessons cancer risks (for several types)
- Lower blood pressure
- Promotes bone health
- Promotes brain health
- Reduces anxiety
- Reduces depression
- Reduces stroke risk
- Weight control

> **Sources**: Mayo Clinic[42], CDC[43], "Physical Activity Guidelines for Americans[44], University of Alberta[45], Department of Biomedical Sciences, University of Missouri[46], Institute for Research in Extramural Medicine, VU University Medical Center[47], Department of Human Movement and Exercise Science, The University of Western Australia[48]

A study released February 2019 in *Neurology* tested whether exercise and dementia risk are related. The researchers concluded: "midlife cognitive and physical activities are independently associated with reduced risk of dementia and dementia subtypes. The results indicate that these midlife activities may have a role in preserving cognitive health in old age[49]."

Another study released in the *Journal of Clinical Pathology* studied 7501 senior citizens over nine years. "Regular exercise was associated with decreased risk of dementia," said lead author Zi Zhou. "Policy-makers should develop effective public health programs and build exercise-friendly environments for the general public[50]."

A longitudinal population study followed 1,462 women over 42 years to measure physical activity's relation to dementia and found those who exercised lowered their dementia risks by 88 percent. Study first author Helena Hörder, professor, Department of Psychiatry and Neurochemistry, University of Gothenburg in Sweden explained the results.

"Our findings indicate that high cardiovascular fitness in midlife is associated with decreased risk of dementia," said Hörder. "Improved cardiovascular fitness in midlife might be a modifiable factor to delay or prevent dementia[51]."

Did the results surprise the researchers?

"I was not surprised that there was an association," said Hörder. "but I was surprised that it was such a strong association between the group with highest fitness and decreased dementia risk[52]."

University of Cambridge researchers released a 10-year study in *Lancelot* and determined exercise can cut dementia risks by a third[53]. Professor Carol Brayne, Cambridge Institute of Public Health, University of Cambridge, served as the lead author. "Although there is no single way to prevent dementia, we may be able to take steps to reduce our risk of developing dementia at older ages. We know what many of these factors are, and that they are often linked," said Brayne. "Simply tackling physical inactivity, for example, will reduce levels of obesity, hypertension and diabetes, and prevent some people from developing dementia as well as a healthier old age in general – it's a win-win situation."

Pointers

The National Institute of Health's "Physical Activity Guidelines for Americans" recommend the following[54]:

- "Move more, sit less"
- Any physical activity is better than none
- Exercise a minimum of 2 ½ hours per week of moderate-intensity exercise, or 1 hour and 14 minutes of vigorous-intensity exercises
- Gain additional benefits by going beyond the minimum amount
- Spread exercise across the week (avoid consecutive off days)
- Do resistance exercises for muscle-building 2-4 days per week

If you suffer a chronic medical condition limiting your physical ability, do what you can. No matter our physical condition, each of us must push ourselves to do what we can and keep increasing our potential. As professor Brayne said, exercise is a "win-win situation." The more we exercise, the stronger we become, and nature keeps raising the bar.

As the NIH suggests, "move more, sit less." Did you know sitting too much can be deadly? Modern humans sit too much, which is why sitting earns its own section.

The question is not if but how we should exercise. Let's review several great options.

Walking

Our ancestors walked wherever they went. There were no cars, subways, elevators, escalators, sitting-jobs, and other luxuries costing us our necessary steps per day.

Then came the horse and buggy, trains, early elevators, and by 1913 the Model T. From there, humans have been working night and day to avoid walking.

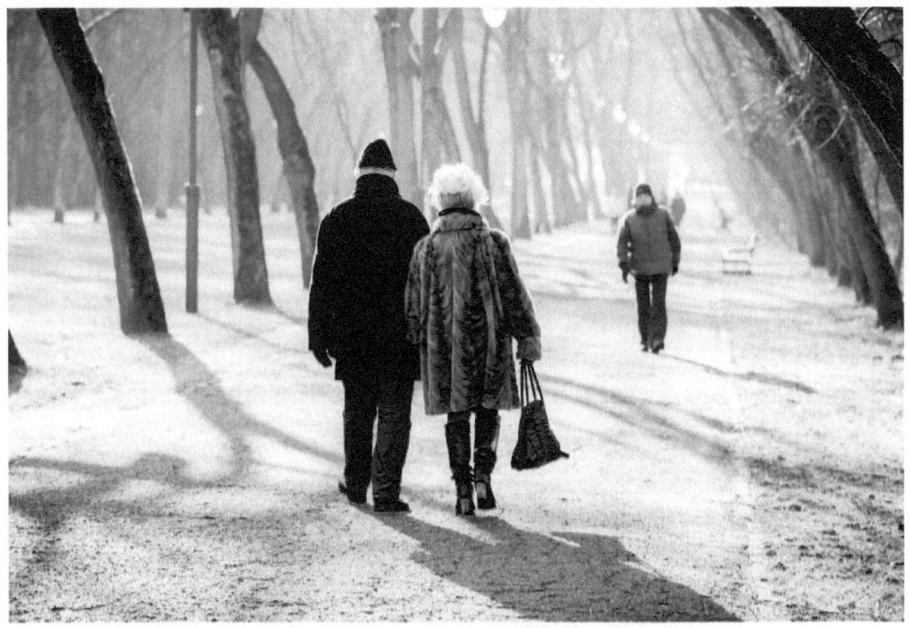

Go for walks!

An Annals of Internal Medicine study found who walked[55] three or more times per week decreased their dementia risk by 38% compared to those who did not exercise[56].

Another study published in Journal of Neurology formed four groups:

1. Group One ate a DASH[57] diet (Dietary Approaches to Stop Hypertension).

2. Group Two exercise, but received no special diet instruction. Supervised exercise included 10 minutes warming up and 35 minutes walking.
3. Group Three adopted the DASH diet and participated in the walking program.
4. The fourth group received a thirty-minute cardiovascular instruction over the phone, but did not exercise or change their diets.

Study lead author James Blumenthal, Duke University clinical psychologist explained their findings. "Our operating model was that by improving cardiovascular risk, you're also improving neurocognitive functioning," said Blumenthal. "You're improving brain health at the same time as improving heart health."

The researchers found Group Three, those who adopted the Dash diet and participated in the exercise group achieved the greatest benefits. Next best, Group Two that participated in the exercise program without any diet changes.

Richard Isaacson, Director of Alzheimer's Prevention Clinic[58], Weill Cornell Medicine[59], weighed in on the study.

"The results showed that controlled aerobic activity within a very short period of time can have a significant impact on the part of the brain that keeps people taking care of themselves, paying their bills and the like," said Isaacson. "Not only can you improve, but you can improve within six months!"

What we do today affects our future physical and cognitive health. "You can do something today for a better brain tomorrow," said Isaacson.

Walk in nature, breathe fresh air, enjoy nature, absorb vitamin D, and reduce your risks for dementia and other life-threatening diseases. Walk several times per week and achieve a healthier, happier version of you.

Running

If you are healthy enough, running pumps the heart, clears the lungs, and strengthens our muscles and internal organs.

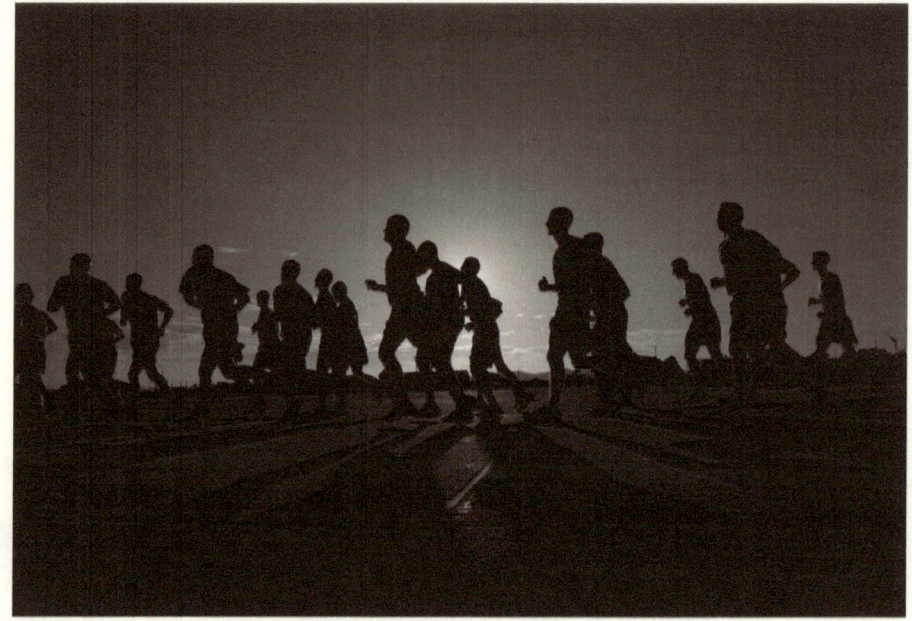

Run by yourself or with others!

You can run by yourself, with a partner, or group, but do so 3-5 times per week.

Remember to stretch before and after. Dress in the right running shoes and apparel. Take water.

A *Journal of Alzheimer's Disease* study followed 154,000 runners and walkers for 11 years. The researchers concluded those who run 7.7-15.3 miles per week reduced dementia risks by 25 %, while those who ran 15 miles or more per week reduced risks by 40 percent[60].

If you are able, run. Physically and cognitively, running extends your quality-of-life.

Hiking

Hiking is a terrific option to get exercise and explore nature. Avoid danger, and consult a doctor if you have any health issues, but there are dozens of hiking options within a short driving distance of most everywhere.

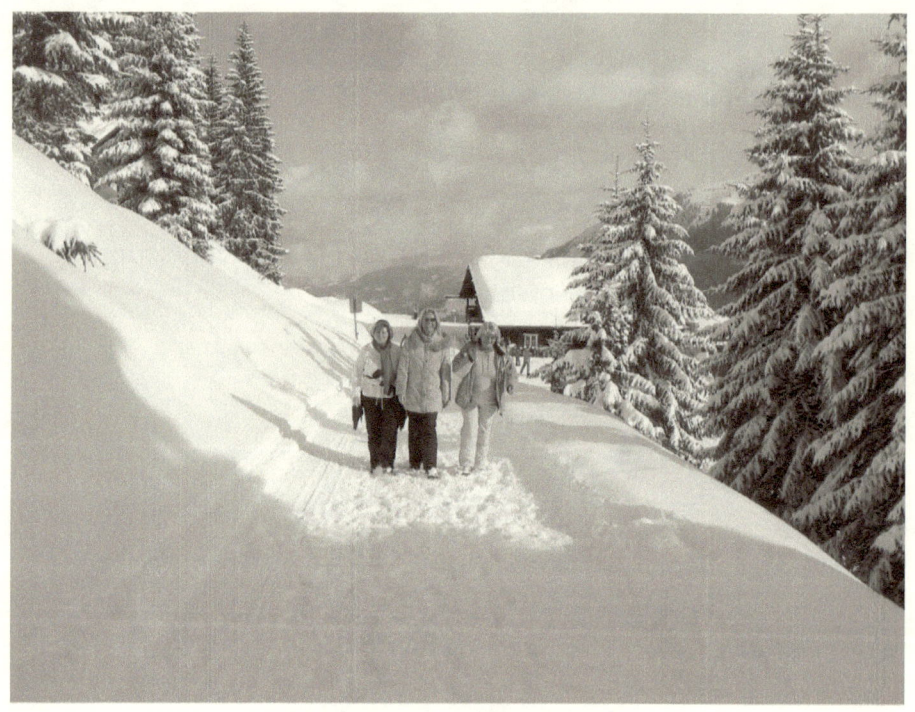

Go hiking with friends!

Whatever hiking you can handle, go for it!

Swimming

If available, swimming is a fantastic regular exercise.

If you do not have another option, become a member of the YMCA or another local club, and go 5-7 days per week. The swimming will strengthen your body and provide endless hours of fun.

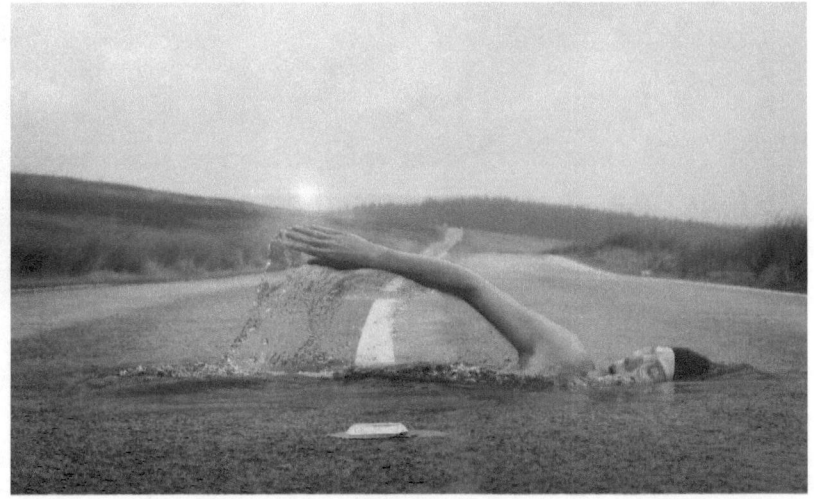

Swim!

I chose physical activities a person can do alone or with another person.

Tennis and other sports are great but require partners. If you choose such a sport, set up backup partners for when your partner is sick, out of town, etc.

Avoid depression

As we covered in early chapters, research connects depression to dementia, but researchers are uncertain whether as a cause or symptom.

Either way, we need to reduce depression. It disrupts our cognitive health and makes us more susceptible to dozens of medical conditions.

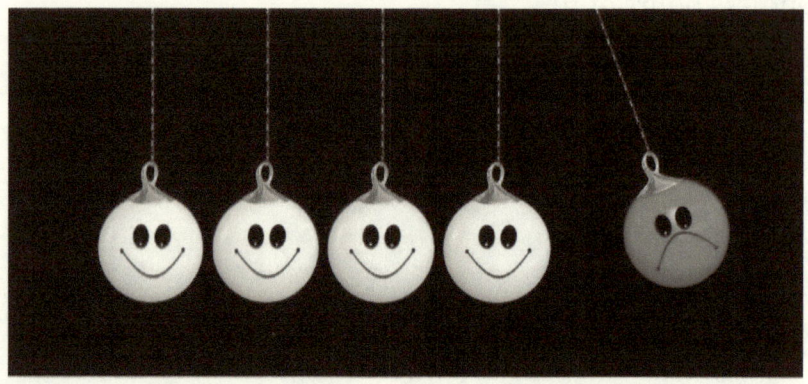

Keep the smile and stop depression!

Researchers from the Department of Neurology, Genetics Program, Boston University designed a "cross-sectional, family-based, case-control" study including 1,953 people with Alzheimer's disease and 2,093 of their relatives who did not have Alzheimer's. Robert C. Green[61], MD, MPH, Harvard Medical School served as the project's lead author.

"Depression symptoms before the onset of AD are associated with the development of AD, even in families where first depression symptoms occurred more than 25 years before the onset of AD," said Green. "These data suggest that depression symptoms are a risk factor for later development of AD[62].

A National Institute of Health sponsored longitudinal

study followed 1,239 older people for 24.7 years to determine if depression increased dementia risk. "Our findings support the hypothesis that depression is a risk factor for dementia and suggest that recurrent depression is particularly pernicious," said the researchers. "Preventing the recurrence of depression in older adults may prevent or delay the onset of dementia[63]."

As covered in the risk factors section, we need more studies to determine the exact link. Depression may cause dementia, or it might be an early symptom. Whatever the relationship to dementia, depression is torturous in the moment, and creates long-term health risks.

Depression demands diligence. Help yourself as much as possible but seek help if required. Navigate to places and people who make you happy, and when possible avoid people and places that depress and make you sad.

People and places are not the only causes of depression. There are many physical, hormonal, and neurological possibilities.

As covered in earlier chapters, we must view depression and mental illnesses for the serious medical condition they are. Seek professional help if required. There is no more shame in seeking medical help for what troubles us emotionally or cognitively than for a broken bone or flu symptoms.

Don't smoke

Do not smoke!

Among the zillion reasons not to smoke is it increases your risk 100% responsible for some vascular dementias, and is directly or indirectly linked to all 16 dementias.

Researchers from the Centre for Mental Health Research, Australian National University conducted a meta-analysis study of 19 prospective studies. The research team concluded: "elderly smokers have increased risks of dementia and cognitive decline[64]."

A team of Finland researchers examined a "prospective data from a multiethnic population-based cohort" including 21,123 people to determine the smoking's impact on dementia. In their conclusions, the team said: "heavy smoking in midlife was associated with a greater than 100% increase in risk of dementia, AD, and VaD more than 2 decades later. These results suggest that the brain is not immune to long-term consequences of heavy smoking[65]."

Several other studies also link smoking to dementia. While we need more studies to determine if smoking directly or indirectly causes dementia, we know it causes a number of medical conditions that increase one's dementia risk.

If you don't smoke, don't start. If you smoke, quit. There is not one good reason to consume tobacco products, but a million sound reasons not to avoid or kick the nasty habit.

More Reasons You Should Not Smoke or Use Tobacco Products

- Ciagarettes include over 7,000 chemicals, over 70 linked to cancer
- Each day, over 3,200 children under 18 light their first cigarette
- Each year, over 41,000 Americans die from second-hand smoke.
- Each year, tobacco costs Americans $332 billion in lost productivity and health care costs
- Over 16 million Americans live with tobacco-caused medical conditions
- Science links tobacco to bronchitis, cancer (several types), chronic airway obstruction, emphysema, erectile dysfunction, eye diseases, immune system deterioration, strokes, rheumatoid arthritis, tuberculosis, and type-2 diabetes
- Tobacco-related illness costs Americans $170 billion each year
- Tobacco kills one of five people in the United States
- Tobacco kills over 7 million people worldwide each year
- Tobacco kills almost 500,000 Americans each year
- Tobacco use robs ten years from the average smoker's life
- The leading cause of preventable deaths is tobacco in the United States and World

Sources: American Lung Association[66], CDC[67], WHO[68], New England Journal of Medicine[69], Federal Trade Commission[70], Department of Neurology, University Hospital

School of Medicine[71], Comprehensive Cardiovascular Center,
Saint Vincent Catholic Medical Centers of New York[72],
FDA/CDC Joint Study[73]

Avoid anxiety

As with depression, scientists do not know if anxiety is a cause or a symptom, but either way you should take steps to avoid or limit anxiety.

According to the American Psychological Association[74], Anxiety is "an emotion characterized by feelings of tension, worried thoughts and physical changes like increased blood pressure[75]."

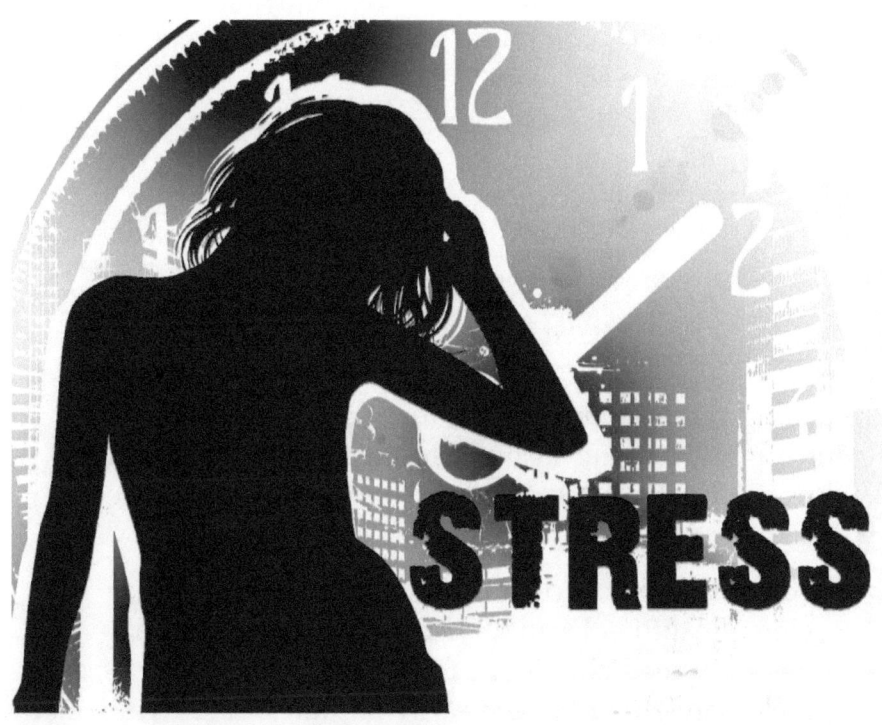

Minimize stress to avoid anxiety.

Premature Aging

Researchers from Brigham and Women's Hospital studied anxiety's affect on the brain. "Many people wonder about whether--and how--stress can make us age faster," said lead author Olivia Okereke. "So, this study is notable for showing a connection between a common form of psychological stress--phobic anxiety--and a plausible mechanism for premature aging."

Funded in part by Harvard Medical, Okereke and the other researchers viewed blood samples from 5,243 women age 42-69 in a nurse's health study. Okereke and the team found anxiety caused the brain to premature age six years[76].

If stress causes premature brain aging and shortens telomeres, are there positive steps to accomplish the opposite?

According to UCSF[77], we can reduce stress, opening more blood flow to the brain, and lengthen our minimize aging through health habits advocated in this chapter. Researchers from UCSF and the Preventive Medicine Research Institute[78]."

Founder and president of the Preventive Medicine Research Institute, Dean Ornish[79], MD, UCSF clinical professor of medicine spoke for the group. "Our genes, and our telomeres, are not necessarily our fate," said Ornish. "So often people think 'Oh, I have bad genes, there's nothing I can do about it. But these findings indicate that telomeres may lengthen to the degree that people change how they live. Research indicates that longer telomeres are associated with fewer illnesses and longer life[80]."

A Canadian study published in the American Journal of Geriatric Psychiatry[81] gauged whether anxiety increases Alzheimer's and dementia symptoms. The research team reviewed cognitive changes every six months and found mild anxiety increased Alzheimer's risks by 33%, moderate anxiety by 78%, and severe anxiety by 135% or more[82].

Another study released in *Frontiers in Neuroscience*[83] followed 5,230 people for ten years, checking them every two years to determine anxiety's relation to dementia. Their findings backed other studies concluding anxiety increases dementia risks[84].

A *JAMA Psychiatry*[85] study focused 54 months on multi-center facilities treating Alzheimer's evaluating anxiety's relationship to cognitive decline in AD patients.

Lead author Robert Pietrzak[86], PhD, MPH, Associate Professor of Psychiatry and Public Health, U.S. Department of Veterans Affairs National Center for PTSD[87] summarized their findings.

"The results of our study suggest that among older adults with a positive beta-amyloid scan, those with elevated anxiety symptoms show a more rapid decline in global cognition, verbal memory, language, and executive function over a 54-month period," said Pietrzak. "This suggests that increased levels of anxiety increase the development of the symptoms of Alzheimer's disease. Thus, assessment, monitoring, and treatment of such symptoms, even subclinical levels, may help inform risk stratification and management of preclinical and prodromal phases of

Alzheimer's disease[88]."

****ONE MORE DEMENTIA LINK*****

Besides anxiety increasing dementia risk, Harvard Medical School[89] warns several anxiety medications increase dementia risk[90].

Benzodiazepines Prescribed for Anxiety that Increase Dementia Risks

- alprazolam (Xanax)
- chlordiazepoxide (Librium)
- clonazepam (Klonopin)
- clorazepate (Tranxene)
- diazepam (Valium)
- flurazepam (Dalmane)
- lorazepam (Ativan)
- oxazepam (Serax)
- paroxetine (Paxil)

National Health Service[91] in Great Britain suggests anxiety and depressions role in dementia risks might be indirect, hypothesizing if one is stressed, suffering anxiety, or depressed, they are less likely to socialize[92] (important in avoiding dementia).

Either way, we should avoid anxiety.

Anxiety and depression also cause high blood pressure and other medical conditions increasing dementia risks, so at minimum there is an indirect link.

To reach anxiety, one must suffer stress first. Minimize stress and avoid anxiety.

Stop raging at every irresponsible driver. Do not torture yourself over things that might happen when you know such worries almost come true. Do not confront every person who deserves a tongue-lashing.

I am not suggesting you become a pushover but knowing when to fight and when not to is an art one must learn to avoid stress.

Stress kills. Do not allow it to kill you!

Don't abuse alcohol

If you care about your health, you have two alcohol choices:

1. Do not drink alcohol.
2. Do not abuse alcohol.

This is not a goody-goody message, but a legitimate health risk warning.

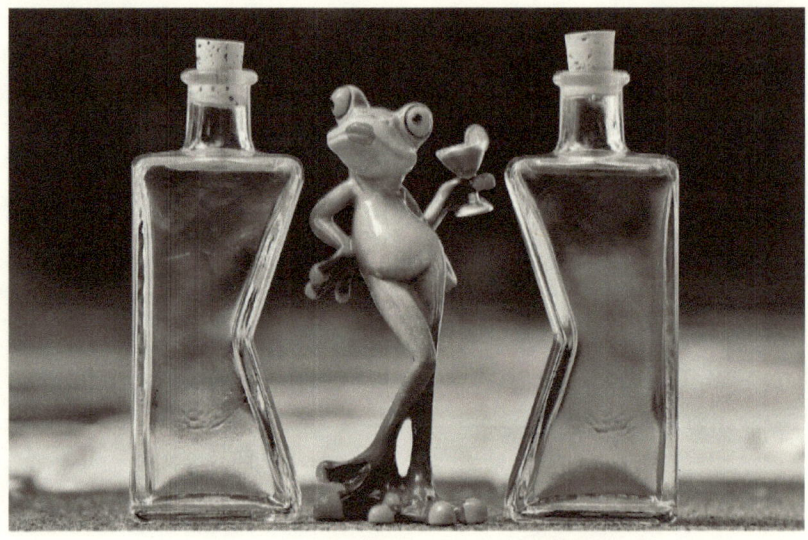

Do not exceed drinking limits!

The limit for women is one beer, a glass of wine, or cocktail per day, no exceptions.

Medical authorities set the limit for men to two beers, glasses of wine, or cocktails, no exceptions.

The rules include occasional drinkers. It does not matter if you limit drinking to once per week, month, or year, do not exceed the daily limit!

Does Alcohol Increase Dementia Risks?

French researchers released a study in Lancet linking alcohol use to an increased dementia risk. The team analyzed 31 million people released from national-wide French hospitals. "Alcohol use disorders were a major risk factor for onset of all types of dementia, and especially early-onset dementia[93]." Heavy drinkers were three times more likely to get dementia than those who did not abuse alcohol. They also found fifty percent of early-onset dementia was alcohol-related.

While the research was exclusive to the French population, 31 million people is a large sample size.

A group of Canadian researchers examined 28 systematic review published in PsycINFO, Embase, and Medline between 2000 and 2017 and concluded: "Heavy alcohol use was associated with changes in brain structures, cognitive impairments, and an increased risk of all types of dementia[94]."

Avoid the madness of alcohol abuse!

Don't demand or expect prescription drugs for every symptom. Ask questions about side effects

Not only can prescription drugs increase one's Parkinson's and dementia risks, but the list of other potential side effects are far greater than the benefits.

Anybody who watches television in the United States if forgiven if their heads spin when the drug commercials spend most the commercial listing the potential side effects.

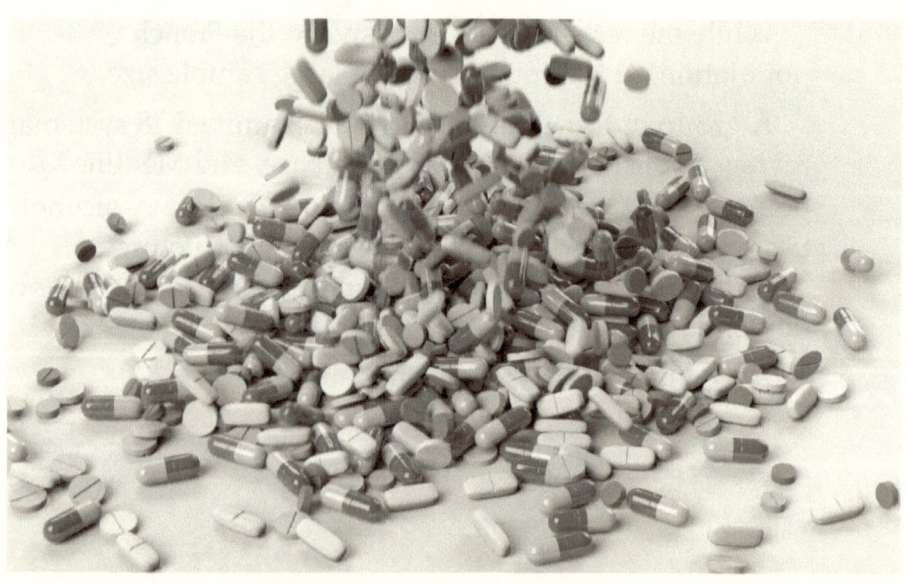

The average American consumes far too many prescription and over-the-counter drugs, often causing far worse medical problems than they are trying to solve.

The United States government has conducted an unsuccessful war for decades against illegal drugs, but legal drugs kill far more people.

Follow the Golden Rule

This is not a religious but spiritual statement: The best way to avoid stress and anxiety is to follow the Golden Rule. The golden rule is the best recipe to achieve happiness, friendship, lasting love, and to evolve throughout one's life.

When we treat others with kindness, we launch positive waves across our species.

The norm is if a person treats us kind, we respond likewise.

Or, if a person mistreats us, we respond from hurt, anger, or frustration.

Break the norm! Be the person who treats others kind and sets a high bar for humanity.

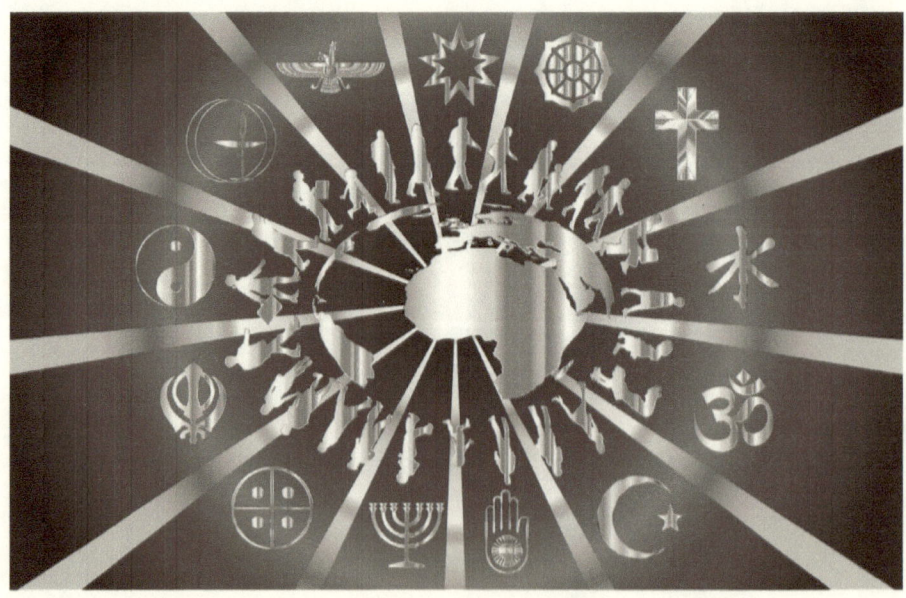

Follow the Golden Rule!

The world has too many preachers and not enough people following the Golden Rule. Follow the Golden Rule and use your live to make the world better.

Laugh when you can

Nothing fights depression, stress, and anxiety like laughter. When others give you reason to laugh, laugh. When they do not, search for the humor in every situation and make yourself laugh.

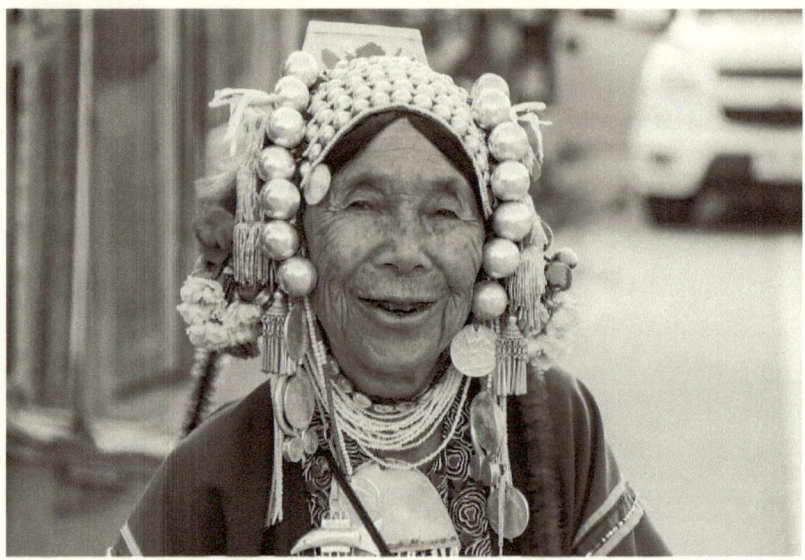

Laugh!

Make it a point to befriend people who make you laugh without hurting others.

Instead of seeing the worse in every situation; search for laughter like a comedian.

Spread laughter and you will be happier and healthier.

Avoid negativity

Negativity is the opposite of laughter, increasing stress, anxiety, and depression.

Two rules:

1. Avoid negative people.
2. Do not be a negative person.

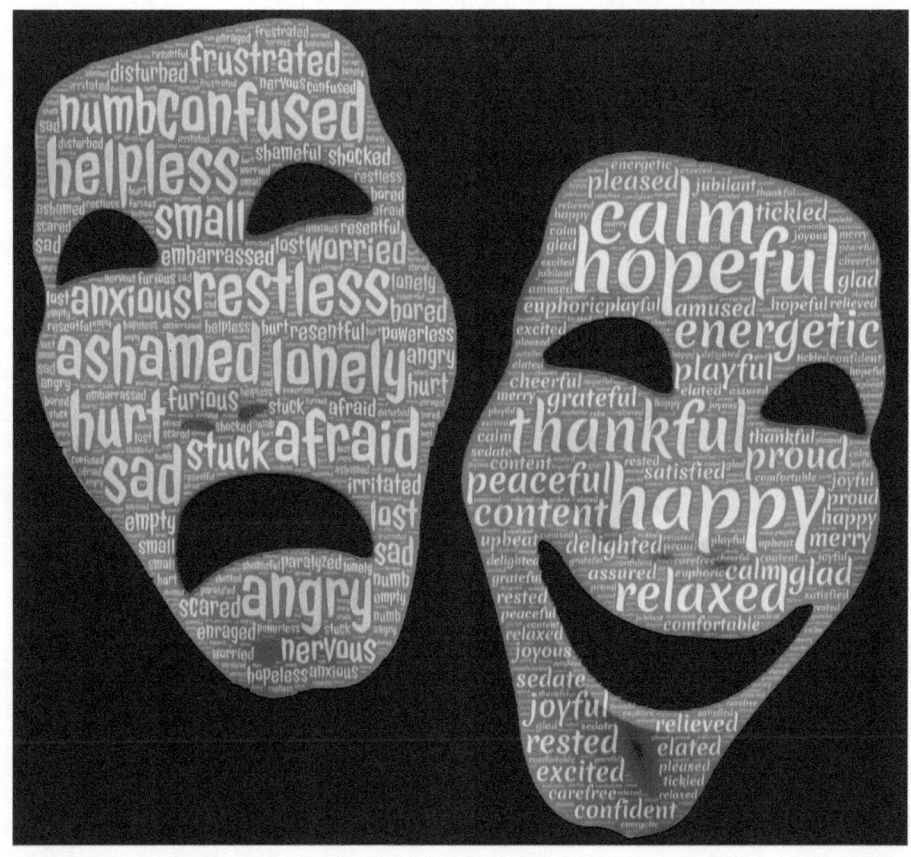

Manage cholesterol and blood pressure

In the chapters *Risk Factors*, *Symptoms*, *Diagnosis*, and *Stages*, we showed that high cholesterol and high blood pressure increase the risk of Parkinson's disease and dementia with Lewy bodies.

High Cholesterol

Unhealthy eating habits causes most people's high cholesterol.

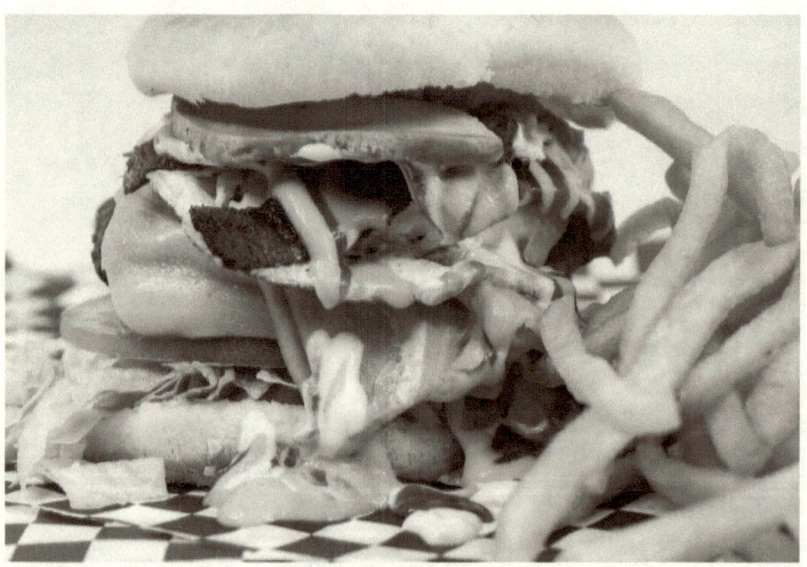

Not the meal of champions!

Eat food high in good cholesterol (HDL) and avoid bad cholesterol (LDL) to avoid or cure high cholesterol.

HDL (good) cholesterol absorbs HDL (bad) cholesterol and transport it to the liver, which will dispose of it[95].

Let's list some LDL and HDL foods, starting with the bad list.

Foods high in LDL (bad) cholesterol

- Dairy
- Trans fats

Foods high in HDL (good) cholesterol

- Beans and legumes
- Whole grains
- Fresh fruit
- Olive oil
- Avocados
- Tempeh
- Unfried Salmon (wild caught fatty fish)
- Red wine (Only 1 for women or 2 for men)
- Flax or Chia seeds
- Nuts

High Blood Pressure

Most people can avoid or fix blood pressure without medication. Not that you should stop taking medication your doctor prescribed, but high blood pressure is another medical condition a healthy lifestyle can avoid or fix. Work out a plan with your doctor.

Most get high blood pressure because we do not eat right, do not exercise, carry unhealthy body fat (the worst being abdominal fat), and otherwise do not take care of ourselves.

If we feed automobiles the wrong liquids in place of oil and gasoline, the infraction destroys the engine.

Why should it be different if we feed our bodies the wrong food?

Socialize

Positive social environments are healthy and reduce our risk of dementia.

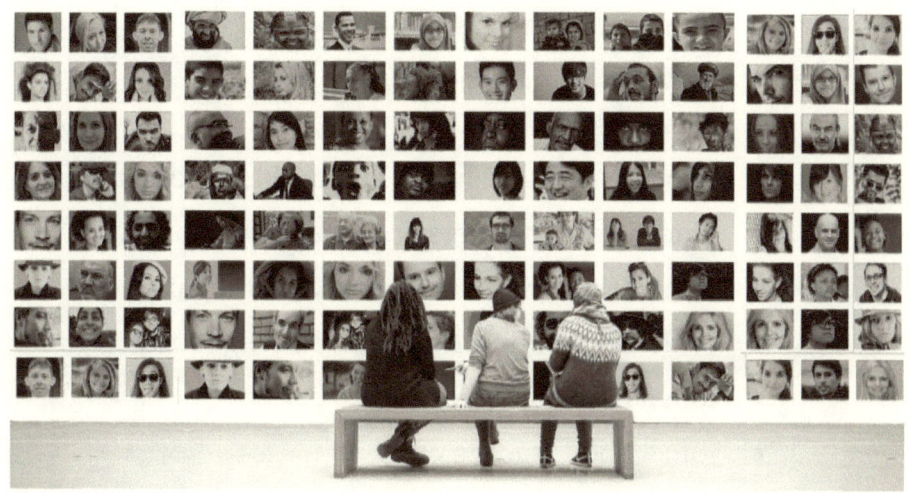

Do you engage regular socialization?

People who do not socialize increase their risk for the dementias whereas regular socializers decrease theirs.

By socialize, we do not mean hang out with people and drink yourself silly, do drugs, eat large portions of unhealthy food, or otherwise increase your risks of all diseases.

Engage in positive social functions:

- Become a community volunteer (also good for the soul)

- If you play a musical instrument, teach a few students
- If you do not play a musical instrument, take lessons
- Take a community college class or two
- Join an arts and crafts club
- Take art lessons and develop skills you can use every day
- Join a walking, jogging, swimming, or other club.
- Find several partners and play chess daily
- Invite friends over for a weekly card game
- Walk the neighborhood and be neighborly
- Join a bowling team
- Join a book reading club!
- Host a weekly dinner
- Organize picnics
- Join an astronomy club and study the stars
- Take a dancing class
- Coach or help coach kids (does not matter what sport)
- Constant visits to the local library (still a treasure!)

There are many regular social environments that inspire laughter, creativity, friendship, and a connectivity healthy humans require.

View your local options and pick the social engagements matching your likes and become a regular contributing member. Be the person you want those around you to be!

CONCLUSION

Congratulations! You have reached the last chapter of *LATE*

Please remember the book is not a finished product, and I will update it as science unfolds more information about this new dementia pathway.

While you might need to reread the guide or refer to certain sections, the book taught:

- you need the right doctor.
- how to describe LATE.
- TDP-43 protein misfolding causes LATE.
- the difference between LATE and Alzheimer's disease.
- known risk factors.
- symptoms in different stages.
- how doctors diagnose LATE.
- how doctors and therapists treat LATE.
- possible ways to reduce the risks or slow LATE.

Please email or call your politicians and ask for better funding for independent research. Tell them your family's story. Remind them how many Americans and humans suffer these awful dementia-causing diseases. Ask them how many unknown dementias are being misdiagnosed like LATE for Alzheimer's all those decades. As taxpayers, we must force our politicians to fund independent dementia research with the same enthusiasm they reward cronies.

Those suffering these diseases cannot fight the fight, so the rest of us must engage and battle for them.

Doctor Hodes, workgroup cochair emphasized research has gotten this far because of, "those who are willing to donate brain tissue after death."

We are grateful for organ donors and their families, as well as all clinical trial participants, who truly are crucial to furthering discoveries that can lead to treatments and cures.--Richard J. Hodes, M.D.

Each of us can make a difference, big or small, in life and death.

Updates

As science advances, so will this book. I update my health books at least once per year, so watch out for Amazon alerts.

Since LATE is a new classified path to dementia, I expect:

- government and private organizations to fund LATE research.
- a steady release of LATE studies, progressing from animal to human studies.
- better diagnosis tools.
- better treatment options.
- greater and continuous scientific discoveries of LATE's causes, symptoms, risk factors, diagnosis tooks, treatment, prevention, and—hopefully one day—a cure.

I will update this book once or twice before the more significant annual update.

Starter To-do List for Somebody and Family once Diagnosed with Dementia.

The person with dementia, loved ones, and family must address several matters early in the disease, including:

- **Care:** Family, loved ones, and dementia patient must make difficult decisions concerning if somebody can become the primary volunteer caregiver. While dementia patients do not require 24/7 care in the early stage, it becomes necessary in middle to late stages.

- **Financial decisions:** There are significant financial decisions to make, and earlier the better. Such a disease becomes a hardship for not only the patient, but also their family. The demands, financial and otherwise, on voluntary caregivers often is devastating. Make difficult financial decisions early.

- **Living Quarters:** While most dementia patients maintain independence in stage one, at some point they require help with daily tasks. Will somebody move in with her or him? Does the patient move in with somebody else? Will it become necessary for him or her to move into an assisted living community in later stages?

- **Living Will**: It is crucial to document dementia patient's wishes while he or she maintains their facilities to make such decisions.

- **Power of Attorney**: It is important to establish a Power of Attorney to empower a trusted loved one to make medical and financial decisions when a patient becomes incapable.

Above is an incomplete list. Once diagnosed, both the person diagnosed and loved ones need to unite and build your own to-do list.

THE END

Of

2019 LATE (The New Dementia)

Please continue for more information and books by Beller Health.

THANK YOU FOR READING

Thank you for reading the entire book. While this is not a literary work to enjoy, I hope you gained useful knowledge of LATE.

If this book benefitted you, please take a moment to share your thoughts in a review. Reader reviews help sell more books and keep producing more!

2019 LATE (The New Dementia) Book Review link =

https://amzn.to/2GV5HL5

Look for annual updates to my health books. I follow new studies and will add any helpful information I find. Health and fitness are top priorities.

I hope you'll develop the habits suggested in this book. Good luck on your health journey. Live long and prosper, my friend.

All the best,

Jerry Beller & Beller Health

OTHER BELLER HEALTH BOOKS

Dementia Risk Factors, Symptoms, Diagnosis, Stages, Treatment, Prevention Series

Alzheimer's Risk Factors & Symptoms

Behavioral Variant Frontotemporal Dementia (bvFTD)

Primary Progressive Aphasia (PPA)

Dementia with Lewy Bodies

Parkinson's disease

Huntington's Disease

Normal Pressure Hydrocephalus

Wernicke-Korsakoff Syndrome

LATE (Limbic-predominant age-related TDP-43 encephalopathy)

ALZHEIMER'S DEMENTIA SERIES

What is Alzheimer's? (2019), book 1

Alzheimer's Risk Factors (2019), book 2

Alzheimer's Symptoms (2019), book 3

Alzheimer's Diagnosis (2019), book 4

Alzheimer's Stages (2019), book 5

How to Prevent & Slow Alzheimer's (2019), book 6

Alzheimer's Treatment (2019), book 7

Other Beller Health Books

Be the Best You!

Dementia Types, Risk Factors, & Symptoms

Alzheimer's Collections

Vascular Dementia (2019)

Lewy Body Dementia (2019)

Frontotemporal Dementia (FTD)

You can view or purchase all Beller Health Books on Amazon at the following web address:

https://amzn.to/2Ub0hRf

ABOUT THE AUTHOR

Beller Health is a team of health researchers and advocates who focus on diseases and cures. Veteran author and researcher Jerry Beller writes accurate medical books in everyday language.

[1] 'LATE Dementia Is a New Type of Brain Disease That Mimics Alzheimer's', *Being Patient*, 2019 <https://www.beingpatient.com/late-dementia/> [accessed 6 May 2019].

[2] 'Guidelines Proposed for Newly Defined Alzheimer's-like Brain Disorder', *National Institute on Aging* <https://www.nia.nih.gov/news/guidelines-proposed-newly-defined-alzheimers-brain-disorder> [accessed 6 May 2019].

[3] 'Nina SILVERBERG', *National Institute on Aging* <https://www.nia.nih.gov/about/staff/silverberg-nina> [accessed 6 May 2019].

[4] 'Richard HODES', *National Institute on Aging* <https://www.nia.nih.gov/about/staff/hodes-richard> [accessed 6 May 2019].

[5] Nina Silverberg, 'The Alzheimer's Disease Centers Program: Updates', 28.

[6] 'Researchers Define Alzheimer's-like Brain Disorder: LATE Symptoms Resembles Alzheimer's Disease but Has Different Cause', *ScienceDaily* <https://www.sciencedaily.com/releases/2019/04/190430121800.htm> [accessed 1 May 2019].

[7] 'New Form of Dementia Discovered, Redefining Mainstream Alzheimer's Science' <https://newatlas.com/new-dementia-disease-late-alzheimers/59491/> [accessed 5 May 2019].

[8] John Gibbs, 'New Type of Dementia Is "100 Times More Common" than ALS', *Medicine News Line*, 2019

<https://medkit.info/2019/05/01/new-type-of-dementia-is-100-times-more-common-than-als/> [accessed 6 May 2019].

9 'Not Too Late to Focus on LATE, an Overlooked Brain Disease', *GEN - Genetic Engineering and Biotechnology News*, 2019 <https://www.genengnews.com/news/prevalent-brain-disease-identified-better-late-than-never/> [accessed 3 May 2019].

10 'Researchers Define Alzheimer's-like Brain Disorder: LATE Symptoms Resembles Alzheimer's Disease but Has Different Cause', *ScienceDaily* <https://www.sciencedaily.com/releases/2019/04/190430121800.htm> [accessed 3 May 2019].

11 'Bart De Strooper Lab' <http://www.vib.be/en/research/scientists/Pages/Bart-De-Strooper-Lab.aspx> [accessed 6 May 2019].

12 'Expert Reaction to a Study Describing a Recently Recognized Alzheimer's-like Brain Disorder | Science Media Centre' <https://www.sciencemediacentre.org/expert-reaction-to-a-study-describing-a-recently-recognized-alzheimers-like-brain-disorder/> [accessed 5 May 2019].

13 'Introducing LATE — A Common TDP-43 Proteinopathy That Strikes After 80 | ALZFORUM' <https://www.alzforum.org/news/research-news/introducing-late-common-tdp-43-proteinopathy-strikes-after-80> [accessed 6 May 2019].

14 Sarah Knapton, 'Hundreds of Thousands with Alzheimer's Are Probably Suffering from Late Disease, Scientists Say', *The Telegraph*, 30 April 2019 <https://www.telegraph.co.uk/science/2019/04/30/hundreds-thousands-alzheimers-probably-suffering-late-disease/> [accessed 5 May 2019].

15 'Researchers Define Alzheimer's-like Brain Disorder', *EurekAlert!* <https://eurekalert.org/pub_releases/2019-04/rumc-rda043019.php> [accessed 3 May 2019].

16 'What Happens to the Brain in Alzheimer's Disease?', *National Institute on Aging* <https://www.nia.nih.gov/health/what-happens-

brain-alzheimers-disease> [accessed 6 May 2019].

[17] 'Stages of Alzheimer's', *Alzheimer's Disease and Dementia* <https://alz.org/alzheimers-dementia/stages> [accessed 6 May 2019].

[18] Peter T. Nelson and others, 'Limbic-Predominant Age-Related TDP-43 Encephalopathy (LATE): Consensus Working Group Report', *Brain* <https://doi.org/10.1093/brain/awz099>.

[19] 'New Dementia Classification for Disease with Alzheimer's like Symptoms', *Alzheimer's Research UK*, 2019 <https://www.alzheimersresearchuk.org/new-dementia-classification-for-disease-with-alzheimers-like-symptoms/> [accessed 6 May 2019].

[20] Allan Adamson, 'New Form Of Dementia LATE Can Be Mistaken As Alzheimer's Disease', *Tech Times*, 2019 <https://www.techtimes.com/articles/242662/20190430/newly-recognized-form-of-dementia-is-sometimes-mistaken-as-alzheimers-how-to-recognize-this-brain-disorder.htm> [accessed 6 May 2019].

[21] 'Researchers Just Found a New Type of Dementia' <http://www.advisory.com/daily-briefing/2019/05/06/alzheimers> [accessed 6 May 2019].

[22] 'When Is "Alzheimer's" Not Alzheimer's? Researchers Characterize a Different Form of Dementia', *ScienceDaily* <https://www.sciencedaily.com/releases/2019/04/190430173210.htm> [accessed 6 May 2019].

[23] 'LATE Dementia Is a New Type of Brain Disease That Mimics Alzheimer's', *Being Patient*, 2019 <https://www.beingpatient.com/late-dementia/> [accessed 6 May 2019].

[24] Genetics Home Reference, 'TARDBP Gene', *Genetics Home Reference* <https://ghr.nlm.nih.gov/gene/TARDBP> [accessed 6 May 2019].

[25] Neuroscience News, 'When Is Alzheimer's Not Alzheimer's? Researchers Characterize a Different Form of Dementia', *Neuroscience News*, 2019 <https://neurosciencenews.com/dementia-tdp-43-late-12090/> [accessed 7 May 2019].

[26] Peter T. Nelson and others, 'Limbic-Predominant Age-Related

TDP-43 Encephalopathy (LATE): Consensus Working Group Report', *Brain* <https://doi.org/10.1093/brain/awz099>.

27 Nelson and others, 'Limbic-Predominant Age-Related TDP-43 Encephalopathy (LATE)'.

28 'When Is Alzheimer's Not Alzheimer's? Researchers Characterize a Different Form of Dementia' <https://medicalxpress.com/news/2019-04-alzheimer-characterize-dementia.html> [accessed 7 May 2019].

29 'Experts Draft Guidelines for Alzheimer's-like Condition', *Medical News Today* <https://www.medicalnewstoday.com/articles/325080.php> [accessed 7 May 2019].

30 'Researchers Just Found a New Type of Dementia'.

31 'Guidelines Proposed for Newly Defined Alzheimer's-like Brain Disorder', *National Institute on Aging* <https://www.nia.nih.gov/news/guidelines-proposed-newly-defined-alzheimers-brain-disorder> [accessed 7 May 2019].

32 'Alzheimer's Disease-Related Dementias Summit 2019 - Agenda' <https://meetings.ninds.nih.gov/Home/Agenda/21149> [accessed 7 May 2019].

33 'TARDBP Gene - GeneCards | TADBP Protein | TADBP Antibody' <https://www.genecards.org/cgi-bin/carddisp.pl?gene=TARDBP> [accessed 7 May 2019].

34 'Diagnostic Criteria Proposed for Advanced-Age Proteinopathy', *PracticeUpdate* <http://www.practiceupdate.com/content/diagnostic-criteria-proposed-for-advanced-age-proteinopathy/83146> [accessed 7 May 2019].

35 Nelson and others, 'Limbic-Predominant Age-Related TDP-43 Encephalopathy (LATE)'.

36 'Diagnostic Guidelines Developed for LATE, New Alzheimer-Like Brain Disorder', *Neurology Live* <https://www.neurologylive.com/clinical-focus/diagnostic-guidelines-late-new-alzheimer-like-brain-disorder> [accessed 7 May 2019].

[37] May 1 and 2019 | HealthDay | 0 |, 'Diagnostic Criteria Proposed for Advanced-Age Proteinopathy | Physician's Weekly' <https://www.physiciansweekly.com/diagnostic-criteria-proposed-for-advanced-age-proteinopathy/> [accessed 7 May 2019].

[38] Nelson and others, 'Limbic-Predominant Age-Related TDP-43 Encephalopathy (LATE)'.

[39] Silvia Pozzi and others, 'Virus-Mediated Delivery of Antibody Targeting TAR DNA-Binding Protein-43 Mitigates Associated Neuropathology', *The Journal of Clinical Investigation*, 129.4 (2019), 1581–95 <https://doi.org/10.1172/JCI123931>.

[40] 'Laval University: Hope for a Cure for Lou Gehrig's Disease', *TIMES OF QUEBEC*, 2019 <https://timesofquebec.com/index.php/2019/02/07/laval-university-hope-for-a-cure-for-lou-gehrigs-disease/> [accessed 4 May 2019].

[41] 'Role of Diet and Nutritional Supplements in Parkinson's Disease Progression' <https://www.hindawi.com/journals/omcl/2017/6405278/> [accessed 24 April 2019].

[42] 'Fitness Fitness Basics', *Mayo Clinic* <https://www.mayoclinic.org/healthy-lifestyle/fitness/basics/fitness-basics/hlv-20049447> [accessed 7 May 2019].

[43] 'Physical Activity for a Healthy Weight | Healthy Weight | CDC', 2019 <https://www.cdc.gov/healthyweight/physical_activity/index.html> [accessed 7 May 2019].

[44] Fitness & Nutrition President's Council on Sports, 'Physical Activity Guidelines for Americans', *HHS.Gov*, 2012 <https://www.hhs.gov/fitness/be-active/physical-activity-guidelines-for-americans/index.html> [accessed 7 May 2019].

[45] D. E. Warburton, N. Gledhill, and A. Quinney, 'Musculoskeletal Fitness and Health', *Canadian Journal of Applied Physiology = Revue Canadienne De Physiologie Appliquee*, 26.2 (2001), 217–37.

[46] M. Harold Laughlin, 'Joseph B. Wolfe Memorial Lecture. Physical Activity in Prevention and Treatment of Coronary Disease: The Battle Line Is in Exercise Vascular Cell Biology', *Medicine and Science in Sports and Exercise*, 36.3 (2004), 352–62.

[47] Isabel Ferreira and others, 'Longitudinal Changes in .VO2max: Associations with Carotid IMT and Arterial Stiffness', *Medicine and Science in Sports and Exercise*, 35.10 (2003), 1670–78 <https://doi.org/10.1249/01.MSS.0000089247.37563.4B>.

[48] Andrew Maiorana and others, 'Exercise and the Nitric Oxide Vasodilator System', *Sports Medicine (Auckland, N.Z.)*, 33.14 (2003), 1013–35 <https://doi.org/10.2165/00007256-200333140-00001>.

[49] James A. Mortimer and Yaakov Stern, 'Physical Exercise and Activity May Be Important in Reducing Dementia Risk at Any Age', *Neurology*, 92.8 (2019), 362–63 <https://doi.org/10.1212/WNL.0000000000006935>.

[50] Zi Zhou and others, 'Association between Exercise and the Risk of Dementia: Results from a Nationwide Longitudinal Study in China', *BMJ Open*, 7.12 (2017), e017497 <https://doi.org/10.1136/bmjopen-2017-017497>.

[51] Helena Hörder and others, 'Author Response: Midlife Cardiovascular Fitness and Dementia: A 44-Year Longitudinal Population Study in Women', *Neurology*, 91.16 (2018), 763–763 <https://doi.org/10.1212/WNL.0000000000006350>.

[52] Jacqueline Howard CNN, 'Your Dementia Risk Tied to How Fit You Are', *CNN* <https://www.cnn.com/2018/03/14/health/dementia-risk-fitness-study/index.html> [accessed 8 May 2019].

[53] Sam Norton and others, 'Potential for Primary Prevention of Alzheimer's Disease: An Analysis of Population-Based Data', *The Lancet Neurology*, 13.8 (2014), 788–94 <https://doi.org/10.1016/S1474-4422(14)70136-X>.

[54] 'Executive Summary: Physical Activity Guidelines for Americans, 2nd Edition', 7.

[55] Eric B. Larson and others, 'Exercise Is Associated with Reduced Risk for Incident Dementia among Persons 65 Years of Age and Older', *Annals of Internal Medicine*, 144.2 (2006), 73–81.

[56] Susan Mayor, 'Regular Exercise Reduces Risk of Dementia and Alzheimer's Disease', *BMJ : British Medical Journal*, 332.7534 (2006), 137 <https://www.ncbi.nlm.nih.gov/pmc/articles/PMC1336790/> [accessed 7 May 2019].

57 'What Is the DASH Diet?' <http://dashdiet.org/what-is-the-dash-diet.html> [accessed 7 May 2019].

58 'Alzheimer's Prevention Clinic | Weill Cornell Medicine' <https://weillcornell.org/services/neurology/alzheimers-disease-memory-disorders-program/our-services/alzheimers-prevention-clinic> [accessed 7 May 2019].

59 'Patient Care | Weill Cornell Medicine' <https://weillcornell.org/> [accessed 7 May 2019].

60 Paul T. Williams, 'Lower Risk of Alzheimer's Disease Mortality with Exercise, Statin, and Fruit Intake', *Journal of Alzheimer's Disease*, 44.4 (2015), 1121–29 <https://doi.org/10.3233/JAD-141929>.

61 'Robert C. Green, MD, MPH - Department of Medicine' <http://researchfaculty.brighamandwomens.org/BRIProfile.aspx?id=5921> [accessed 8 May 2019].

62 Robert C. Green and others, 'Depression as a Risk Factor for Alzheimer Disease: The MIRAGE Study', *Archives of Neurology*, 60.5 (2003), 753–59 <https://doi.org/10.1001/archneur.60.5.753>.

63 Vonetta M. Dotson, May A. Beydoun, and Alan B. Zonderman, 'Recurrent Depressive Symptoms and the Incidence of Dementia and Mild Cognitive Impairment', *Neurology*, 75.1 (2010), 27–34 <https://doi.org/10.1212/WNL.0b013e3181e62124>.

64 Kaarin J. Anstey and others, 'Smoking as a Risk Factor for Dementia and Cognitive Decline: A Meta-Analysis of Prospective Studies', *American Journal of Epidemiology*, 166.4 (2007), 367–78 <https://doi.org/10.1093/aje/kwm116>.

65 Minna Rusanen and others, 'Heavy Smoking in Midlife and Long-Term Risk of Alzheimer Disease and Vascular Dementia', *Archives of Internal Medicine*, 171.4 (2011), 333–39 <https://doi.org/10.1001/archinternmed.2010.393>.

66 'Tobacco Facts | State of Tobacco Control', *American Lung Association* <https://www.lung.org/our-initiatives/tobacco/reports-resources/sotc/facts.html> [accessed 8 May 2019].

67 CDCTobaccoFree, 'Fast Facts', *Centers for Disease Control and*

Prevention, 2019
<https://www.cdc.gov/tobacco/data_statistics/fact_sheets/fast_facts/index.ht
m> [accessed 8 May 2019].

[68] 'WHO | WHO Report on the Global Tobacco Epidemic 2017', *WHO*
<http://www.who.int/tobacco/global_report/2017/en/> [accessed 8 May
2019].

[69] Prabhat Jha and others, '21st-Century Hazards of Smoking and
Benefits of Cessation in the United States', *New England Journal of Medicine*,
368.4 (2013), 341–50 <https://doi.org/10.1056/NEJMsa1211128>.

[70] 'Ftc_cigarette_report_2017.Pdf'
<https://www.ftc.gov/system/files/documents/reports/federal-trade-
commission-cigarette-report-2017-federal-trade-commission-smokeless-
tobacco-report/ftc_cigarette_report_2017.pdf> [accessed 8 May 2019].

[71] P. A. Wolf and others, 'Cigarette Smoking as a Risk Factor for Stroke.
The Framingham Study', *JAMA*, 259.7 (1988), 1025–29.

[72] John A Ambrose and Rajat S Barua, 'The Pathophysiology of Cigarette
Smoking and Cardiovascular Disease: An Update', *Journal of the American
College of Cardiology*, 43.10 (2004), 1731–37
<https://doi.org/10.1016/j.jacc.2003.12.047>.

[73] Brian L. Rostron, Cindy M. Chang, and Terry F. Pechacek, 'Estimation of
Cigarette Smoking-Attributable Morbidity in the United States', *JAMA Internal
Medicine*, 174.12 (2014), 1922–28
<https://doi.org/10.1001/jamainternmed.2014.5219>.

[74] 'American Psychological Association (APA)', *Https://Www.Apa.Org*
<https://www.apa.org/index> [accessed 8 May 2019].

[75] 'Anxiety', *Https://Www.Apa.Org*
<https://www.apa.org/topics/anxiety/index> [accessed 8 May 2019].

[76] Olivia I. Okereke and others, 'High Phobic Anxiety Is Related to Lower
Leukocyte Telomere Length in Women', *PLOS ONE*, 7.7 (2012), e40516
<https://doi.org/10.1371/journal.pone.0040516>.

[77] 'Lifestyle Changes May Lengthen Telomeres, A Measure of Cell Aging |
UC San Francisco', *Lifestyle Changes May Lengthen Telomeres, A Measure of
Cell Aging | UC San Francisco*
<https://www.ucsf.edu/news/2013/09/108886/lifestyle-changes-may-

lengthen-telomeres-measure-cell-aging> [accessed 8 May 2019].

[78] Michael T. Lee focus97, 'Preventive Medicine Research Institute', *Preventive Medicine Research Institute* <http://www.pmri.org> [accessed 8 May 2019].

[79] 'Lifestyle Changes May Lengthen Telomeres, A Measure of Cell Aging | UC San Francisco'.

[80] 'Lifestyle Changes May Lengthen Telomeres, A Measure of Cell Aging | UC San Francisco'.

[81] 'American Psychological Association (APA)'.

[82] Linda Mah, Malcolm A. Binns, and David C. Steffens, 'Anxiety Symptoms in Amnestic Mild Cognitive Impairment Are Associated with Medial Temporal Atrophy and Predict Conversion to Alzheimer Disease', *The American Journal of Geriatric Psychiatry*, 23.5 (2015), 466–76 <https://doi.org/10.1016/j.jagp.2014.10.005>.

[83] 'Frontiers in Neuroscience' <https://www.frontiersin.org/journals/neuroscience> [accessed 8 May 2019].

[84] Marion Mortamais and others, 'Anxiety and 10-Year Risk of Incident Dementia—An Association Shaped by Depressive Symptoms: Results of the Prospective Three-City Study', *Frontiers in Neuroscience*, 12 (2018) <https://doi.org/10.3389/fnins.2018.00248>.

[85] 'JAMA Network | Home of JAMA and the Specialty Journals of the American Medical Association' <https://jamanetwork.com/> [accessed 8 May 2019].

[86] 'Robert Pietrzak, PhD, MPH > Psychiatry | Yale School of Medicine' <https://medicine.yale.edu/psychiatry/people/robert_pietrzak-2.profile> [accessed 8 May 2019].

[87] 'Clinical Neurosciences PTSD Research Program > Psychiatry | Yale School of Medicine' <https://medicine.yale.edu/psychiatry/research/programs/clinical_peo ple/ptsd.aspx> [accessed 8 May 2019].

[88] Amy Gimson and others, 'Support for Midlife Anxiety Diagnosis as an Independent Risk Factor for Dementia: A Systematic Review', *BMJ Open*, 8.4

(2018), e019399 <https://doi.org/10.1136/bmjopen-2017-019399>.

89 Harvard Health Publishing, 'Health Information and Medical Information', *Harvard Health* <https://www.health.harvard.edu/> [accessed 8 May 2019].

90 Harvard Health Publishing, 'Two Types of Drugs You May Want to Avoid for the Sake of Your Brain', *Harvard Health* <https://www.health.harvard.edu/mind-and-mood/two-types-of-drugs-you-may-want-to-avoid-for-the-sake-of-your-brain> [accessed 8 May 2019].

91 'Home', *Nhs.Uk*, 2018 <https://www.nhs.uk/> [accessed 8 May 2019].

92 'Can Dementia Be Prevented?', *Nhs.Uk*, 2017 <https://www.nhs.uk/conditions/dementia/dementia-prevention/> [accessed 8 May 2019].

93 Michaël Schwarzinger and others, 'Contribution of Alcohol Use Disorders to the Burden of Dementia in France 2008–13: A Nationwide Retrospective Cohort Study', *The Lancet Public Health*, 3.3 (2018), e124–32 <https://doi.org/10.1016/S2468-2667(18)30022-7>.

94 Jürgen Rehm and others, 'Alcohol Use and Dementia: A Systematic Scoping Review', *Alzheimer's Research & Therapy*, 11.1 (2019), 1 <https://doi.org/10.1186/s13195-018-0453-0>.

95 CDC, 'LDL and HDL Cholesterol: "Bad" and "Good" Cholesterol', *Centers for Disease Control and Prevention*, 2017 <https://www.cdc.gov/cholesterol/ldl_hdl.htm> [accessed 24 April 2019].

www.ingramcontent.com/pod-product-compliance
Lightning Source LLC
Chambersburg PA
CBHW021835170526
45157CB00007B/2807